Meditation

The Journey Beyond The Mind

Table of Contents

Preface

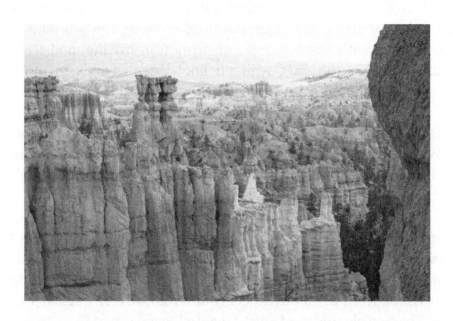

It's the 21st century. We stand at the boundary of the past and the future. Scientifically, we now know more about the world than we have ever known before. But because of the blistering pace of technological change, the shape of the future's horizon is a mystery. We don't know what the world will be like in one hundred years. We can only be certain that it won't be like it is now.

One of the most noteworthy trends of recent years is the way techniques of meditation, mindfulness, and yoga have burst into the mainstream. Though they come from ancient religions, scientific research touts their benefits. But with the current state of scientific knowledge, many of us find it hard to accept the ancient dogmas that come with these techniques. We hunger for something more nutritious than McMindfulness – but at the same time, we find it impossible to swallow the old religious certainties of a bygone era.

It seems like a long time ago when I first set down on the spiritual path. I was just out of college, and I was experiencing a spiritual crisis. The uncertainty of entering the job market combined with other sources of turmoil in my life, and I felt like I was in the dark with no knowledge of how to move forward and no light to guide me.

During this time I developed an interest in spiritual ideas. What brought this on was a series of unusual dreams. But since there's nothing more boring than hearing someone else's dreams, I'll spare you the tedious details.

In any case, I started to experiment with many different ways of getting in touch with the source, but the one that stuck was meditation. I did meditation for years without actually seeing anything from it. In retrospect, I don't know why I stuck with it. I had no clear idea of what I wanted to get out of it.

Perhaps that was for the best. Slowly – very slowly, it seemed, at first – the darkness lifted from my mind. Where before I had felt only confusion and despair, I began to experience hope and elation in the smallest things – a patch of golden sunlight falling on green grass, the soft sound of rain against a window pane.

As I gained more familiarity with this openness, I realized that this was a significant moment. I had struck a rich vein within myself and found gold.

Nothing changed in my outer circumstances to precipitate this discovery. But because of some strange persistence on my part, I had kept rubbing my mind again and again until a layer of grime came off, and, lo and behold, beneath it was a brightly shining mirror. It reflected everything vividly and precisely. It showed me to myself.

With my newfound sense of freedom and joy, I left my job and set out to discover the world. Without much money in my pocket, I traveled to many different countries, especially in Asia, and slummed it in very cheap hotels and guest houses.

I spent my time reading about different spiritual traditions. I sought out teachers of these traditions and learned from them. Buddhism, Hinduism, Taoism, Sufism – you name it.

I found that, although these traditions differed on many points, on the most essential matters they were in agreement. So I resolved to focus on this essence and cut out the extraneous stuff.

I don't claim to have all the answers to life's most pressing spiritual questions. But what I do have, the discovery that I can offer to you, is very precious. It is a lifeline that connects me to the core of my being. And it can be a lifeline for you too.

It is both the most authentic, most genuine part of myself, and that which allows me to be genuine in the world. Since that day when the fog began to lift from my mind, my life has been a process of going deeper and deeper into my experience of that and allowing it to transform my life from the inside out.

My aim in writing this book is not to convert anyone, but to point you in the most fruitful direction for self-discovery. I was like a miner or archaeologist. I just kept digging and excavating my own mind until I discovered buried treasure.

That is what I want for you, as well. I want to inspire you to take out your shovel and start digging.

It's takes effort and persistence, but when you hit that vein, you'll realize it was worth every effort you put into it.

This book is written for anyone who finds themselves standing at this spiritual crossroads, unsure of which path to take. I have spent years traveling, studying, and practicing different systems, and in this book I will distill the essence of them for you – pared down to the simplest elements, without dogma or religious trappings.

The key theme I will keep sounding is what I call *authentic presence*. What exactly is authentic presence? It is the truest, inmost part of you. And it is the goal of many spiritual systems and practices. Someone who has reached the pinnacle of those paths always lives in authentic presence. They embody it. They *are* it – 24/7. This state is called the awakened state or enlightenment.

Authentic presence has been called by many names – the Self, spirit, consciousness, the divine within, the image of God, buddhanature. But I've chosen the phrase "authentic presence" because it's not so much a *thing* as a *way of being* to yourself and to others. At the same time, it's not just a temporary state, but an abiding reality that you can discover within yourself.

Authentic presence is not about making yourself happy or being a better person. It's about fundamental self-honesty, which allows you to be honest with others. So the goal of this path of authentic presence doesn't have to do with capturing a state of bliss, erasing your negativity, doing an emotional detox, or retreating from the challenges of life. It is, instead, a way of opening yourself up to challenges and negativity so that they can be transformed.

The path of authentic presence could be considered synonymous with the spiritual path. The best way to discover authentic presence within yourself and cultivate that state is through the practice of meditation. This is not a matter of religious dogma. It's simply what has worked for many aspirants for millennia. It is a powerful technique that has withstood the test of time.

Through meditation, it's possible to have a glimpse of authentic presence. That one, brief glimpse inspires confidence in the technique and the path. Then, through further practice, you touch on the experience again and again. You learn to relax, without trying to hold on to anything, which prolongs the experience. Then you are able to bring it into everyday situations, which transforms your life.

But now let's start at the beginning: ourselves, as we are right now.

Chapter 1. The Human Condition

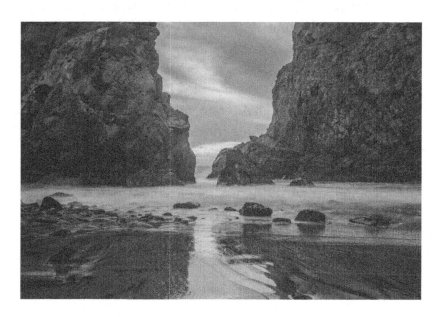

Communicating with Pain

Many philosophers, prophets, and saints have tried to put their finger on the human condition. Some say that there is something fundamentally wrong with us, and we carry around the burden of original sin. Some say that we're fundamentally good, and the negative side of our existence is a temporary situation – a crust of dirt and grime that's built up over time and hides our pure nature.

Whatever the case, they all agree that something is wrong. They share the basic intuition that the human situation is not ideal, but that we could have something better. Some better kind of existence is a genuine possibility for us.

You could say that the point of a spiritual system is to give us a roadmap showing the way from Point A to Point B, along with a few useful techniques to speed us on our journey. But where and what exactly is *Point A*? Like authentic presence, it has also been described in many ways. It is alienation from the divine. It is a fallen state of sin. It is the darkness of ignorance. However we label our situation, the fact is that pain is what clues us into the fact that something is wrong. I'm not talking about the *ouch* kind of pain, like your hand getting hit by a hammer. I'm talking about emotional pain. The pain of loss. The pain of feeling alienated or alone. The pain of thwarted expectations and unfulfilled desires. The pain of worry and stress. The pain of anguish, sadness, irritation, confusion, anger, hatred, disappointment.

This pain is such a fundamental part of our lives that it seems woven into the very nature of things. Many of us just take it for granted that pain is a part of life and never try to do anything about it. Others try to sweep it under the rug, pretend it's not there, and put on a happy face. Still others try to make it go away with different remedies and fixes – anything from medication to meditation.

The path of authentic presence, however, acknowledges the reality of pain and believes it has a lesson to teach. When we pay attention to it and watch it, we can learn about it – what it is, where it comes from, how it distorts our perceptions and affects our mental state – what it *means*.

The path of authentic presence is not about trying to cure or get rid of our pain. Instead, we treat it like a guest. We invite it to sit at our table. We say, "Come in, sit down, have some tea. Let's talk. What's bothering you?"

When we achieve some kind of communication with our pain, we can gain insight into it and effect a transformation. Somehow, just by giving up our struggle with it, the pain becomes less painful. We accept that we might have something to learn from it. That attitude of openness allows genuine insight to take place. Then we can begin to understand how the whole thing fits together. If the mind is like an ecosystem, what is pain's ecological role?

The Egosystem

Painful emotions or states of mind are bound up with what we might call the *egosystem*. The egosystem is an entire complex of mental and emotional habits that is self-sustaining. Once it exists, it takes on a life of its own. It exists just to keep maintaining its existence. That is very circular, but the egosystem rarely stops to question such things. It just keeps churning through emotions and mental states, thoughts and narratives, just to keep itself going, a relentless locomotive. The egosystem is terrified of stopping its perpetual motion.

The egosystem is exactly what we think of when we think *I*-thoughts and *me*-thoughts. The egosystem *is* you – and me. The driving force behind ego is a fundamental sense of insecurity. The movement and energy of living situations are too much. They're just too intense for us. They start to seem like a chaos that will overwhelm us, and we fear getting drowned in them. That leads us to want to grab hold of something solid, to find a fixed point in the chaotic push-and-pull of existence.

This motivating insecurity is like a seed, and the rich soil of our minds gives it the perfect growing conditions. Once the seed is planted, it evolves into a whole thriving, all-consuming organism. It's a weed that takes over the whole garden.

Once the fundamental insecurity takes hold, it grows roots and branches. Ego is sustained by thoughts and beliefs, and mostly these take the form of narratives. We tell ourselves stories

8

about ourselves. These stories define who we are – where we are, where we've been, where we're going, and what kinds of challenges we face on our way there. For the most part, our self-narratives are just convenient fictions. They're not really true, but they're good enough for our purposes.

The problem with these narratives is that they generate a lot of pain. We become preoccupied with the past and the future, so that we are unable to enjoy the present. Have you ever got so lost in thought about your plans, or wandered so far down memory lane, that you became totally unaware of your surroundings? Maybe something jolted you from your reveries and suddenly brought you back to the present moment. You realized you were not really there at all. Your awareness had stepped out of the office and gone on a vacation.

In general, thoughts about the past and future don't bring any satisfaction to us. Many thoughts about the future take the form of worry or anxiety. Or we might fantasize about what we want in the future. In our mind's eye, we might see ourselves getting a promotion, getting the perfect birthday present, watching our favorite team win, or getting the girl or guy of our dreams. Forget the fact that such thoughts might lead to frustration later. Right now, at this moment, they are keeping us from enjoying what we already have. We feel a twang of sadness that we're separate from the object of desire.

Another way the egosystem can create pain for us is anger. We have all sorts of stories and ideas about ourselves. We hold on to many belongings. We make a lot of plans and preparations for the future. The minute someone comes along and threatens those things, anger comes up. Sometimes anger actually achieves its purpose and removes the threat. But most of the time, it just escalates the situation.

Suppose you get into an argument with your spouse or partner. Some conflict comes up, and they are raising their voice at you, anger is flashing in their eyes. The go-to strategy of ego is usually to defend itself, its agenda and priorities. So now, instead of one angry ego, there are two. Both egos feel under attack. Both respond by pushing back with further aggression. In no time, the quarrel reaches a fever pitch. Both of you are speaking words that can't be unspoken and saying hurtful things you don't really mean. Maybe one of you even starts throwing things or getting violent.

Or maybe you just immediately roll over when your significant other quarrels with you. You take a strategy of appeasement. You just retreat and say sorry. But deep inside, you feel pretty rotten about it. Not only did they attack you, but you just surrendered. Your sense of self-respect takes a hit. You feel weak. Maybe you try to get back at them with passive-aggressive actions. You might not have the guts to stand up for yourself when they argue with you, but you can sure make them suffer for it in other ways.

There is a genuine alternative to getting into this toxic predicament. If your awareness is always turned to authentic presence, the slings and arrows others throw at you can't touch you. You might as well try to damage empty space with a bullet.

I can't tell you how to approach such scenarios. There's no rulebook for handling life's situations. It's not about executing a strategy or tactic – that would just be another manipulation, another way of trying to advance your agenda. It's about fundamentally altering your approach by dropping your agenda altogether. In a later chapter we'll talk more about how to work with negative situations through authentic presence.

Dualistic Thought

You've probably heard of nondualism, but for now let's just talk about dualism, which is what we already know. We are already consumed by dualistic thoughts, so their logic must make some sense to us.

It starts with the split between self and other. We have to be very careful here, because when I say "split" it doesn't mean that self and other were some single, shapeless thing before, and then we cut it into pieces. And the "nonduality" of nondualism doesn't refer to a kind of eternal monad hanging out in the sky above us. It doesn't mean the oneness of all things.

Whether the universe is one or not is beside the point. The point is how our habitual patterns of thinking work. And they work by pairing everything off into binary opposites. So you have the ego and the world – or self and other, I and you/he/she/it/they. That's the first pair, the baseline concept that is the foundation for the whole egosystem.

From the perspective of authentic presence, it's all a big self-deception. It's an elaborate con we're playing. We were trying to fool the world, but we got so into it that we forgot it was a ruse, and now we really believe the lie. So we were trying to manipulate something, to protect ourselves, but we ended up setting a trap and falling into it.

We do that by identifying something called the "self," and at first we identify it with our body. Later on we might develop some more complicated twists, and say, well, it's not the body that *I* really am, but the spirit. This is just a more refined kind of self-deception.

On top of the self–other distinction, we build another layer, good and bad. Good and bad really have to do with what benefits *me* – i.e. this ego – and what hurts me. And if it doesn't really help or hurt me, or do anything to me, then it's not interesting to me at all – it's neutral.

And so we also have pleasant and unpleasant, friend and enemy, angel and demon, clean and dirty, and so on. These are the basic building blocks for the whole complicated structure of ego.

Whatever thoughts you have, whatever stories you tell yourself – if you have the guts to take them apart, you'll find that this is what they're made of. These basic concepts are the constituent elements of ego.

All of these concepts all boil down to one thing, and that's protecting ourselves. Protecting ourselves means keeping the game going. Whatever we do, we have to make sure to close all the gaps in our story, or else the whole thing might just fall apart. And then we'll be left with nothing.

But that nothingness is everything. It's infinite. It just keeps going and going. If we allow the con to fall apart, or if we dismantle it carefully, piece by piece, then we can glimpse the nothingness, and then live the nothingness, and finally *be* the nothingness.

If that sounds nihilistic, it's not. Nothingness is not really nothing. But if we try to make it something, if we try to pin it down and say it's this or that, we're just manipulating it and trying to turn it into a comfy home for the ego.

So it's better just to say there's nothing there, but that nothing is everything. If we can actually accomplish *being* that nothing, then the whole world is contained within that.

I hope that doesn't sound too mystical. The seekers of the past who have found authentic presence and lived it have all tried to express something that's outside of ego's frame of reference. To do that, they had to use ego's language.

The trouble is, dualistic language was never intended to express authentic presence; in fact, it was intended to cover it up. So inevitably, they have stumbled into paradox. When we try to pin down the reality of authentic presence, we get into trouble. But there's no paradox in the authentic nature of things.

Styles of Emotion

On one level our emotions seem very organic and healthy. That's not entirely wrong. They're a natural outgrowth of our personality.

But the way we experience them is not so healthy. When we really understand what's going on within us, emotionally, our psychological life – or at least our egoistic interpretation of it – looks very mechanical.

That's because, when we're being inauthentic, the working of our emotions is dictated by the logic of ego. Ego tries to work emotional energy to its advantage. It manipulates that energy and freezes it up into stereotyped responses – the emotions – which become habits. The habits, practiced again and again, become extremely hard to uproot.

The basic engine of most of our emotions is the duality of attraction and aversion. This duality reflects the dualistic thought patterns that give rise to it. Because we have self and other, good and bad, pleasant and painful, approach and retreat, we also have attraction and aversion.

- *Attraction* is the emotional force that pushes us to some object or person. Subjectively, it might feel like a kind of magnetism that the object is working on us, drawing us to it. But that's just a trick we play on ourselves.

   Some object is pleasurable, or we imagine that it will give us pleasure. Maybe the "object" is actually a person. It could be a cupcake or someone we want to sleep with.

   From the standpoint of the emotion itself, it doesn't really matter if it's a thing or a person we want. The character of the emotion is the same any way you slice it.

   We want to possess them or it, whichever the case may be. We want to bring it into our territory and make it our own, so we can sustain that feeling of pleasure. So we advance towards it in order to seize it. That is one kind of game we play.

- *Aversion* is the emotion behind wanting to protect ourselves from something or someone. Or it could be we want to destroy them. Either way, we experience something as a threat and want to neutralize it.

   The specific emotion could be disgust, anger, or something like that. In any case, it's a species of aversion. We have our little patch of ground and want to make sure nothing comes inside that could hurt us.

   We feel disgusted when we see a rotten fruit. We feel angry if someone dings our car in a fender bender. Something sets off the emotion of aversion, which leads to a cascade of thoughts and emotions.

The end result is that we take action. We throw the fruit away in disgust. We jump out of our car and start yelling at the other driver, "What the hell were you doing?" Or maybe we bite our tongue and simmer with resentment on the inside. However we react, the attitude is aggressive and hostile.

There are infinite elaborations of these two emotional poles. Envy is a curious emotion that combines elements of attraction and aversion. We desire what the other person has, while at the same time hating them for having it.

Other styles of emotion are deeply confused. Paranoia is a spin on aversion, except in this case we imagine shadowy threats are working everywhere behind the scenes against us. We create all sorts of delusions from our overactive imagination.

We have resentment, fear, jealousy, suspicion, passion – the list goes on.

But the mechanism of emotion is based on this duality of attraction and aversion. There is a seesaw action to it, which is determined by the logic of dualistic thought itself. There is a self and an other, therefore there is something to enrich and defend, and there is something to be gained – or to defend against.

Opening the Windows

The egosystem isn't just about our thoughts and self-narratives. It also drives us to action. Because of ego, we are constantly playing games, manipulating people and situations to get what we want and get rid of what we don't want. Usually these manipulations are totally opaque to us. We have no idea that we're even doing them, because we don't know what it's like *not* to play ego's games. That's because we don't have an experience of living authentically. We haven't made ourselves familiar with authentic presence.

Ego doesn't give up its habits easily. It goes down kicking and screaming. But when we finally do manage to start giving up our many self-deceptions and manipulations, it comes as a huge relief. It's very raw and personal. At the same time, it's very refreshing. It's as if we had been living in a small, dark, dirty room, breathing the same stale air for ages. Suddenly someone pulls back the curtains and throws open the windows and fresh air comes pouring in. Sunlight fills the room. We realize that there's a reality outside of our dark little room. Not only that, but the world is so much bigger than we thought it was. It's a wide open, full of new and wonderful things. We feel a sense of curiosity and discovery about ourselves and the world.

Ego is very small-minded. It's completely preoccupied with protecting itself, holding its ground, keeping its territory, fending off threats. The mentality of ego is endless claustrophobia.

Authentic presence is wide open and vast. It has nothing to protect or hold on to. It's open, generous, and childlike. It wants to discover and experience. Its fundamental attitude is that life is an unexplored terrain with unknown horizons and limitless potential. While ego is concerned with wrapping itself in a tight cocoon, keeping its defenses up, authentic presence wants to emerge into the daylight.

I have already said that authentic presence is not a cure for pain. And it doesn't come all at once. It's a process. Painful situations still occur. But there are two ways of relating to them. You can relate to them in ego's way, or you can relate to them with authentic presence. If you relate to painful situations with ego, then you'll experience them as a threat, something you need protection from. But somehow, the process of protecting yourself just leads to more pain.

But if you relate to painful situations with authentic presence, each situation becomes a springboard to further discovery and ever fresher possibilities. You emerge unto challenges and situations instead of shrinking from them. And each emergence becomes an opening up. It widens the vistas of life.

Chapter 2. Being

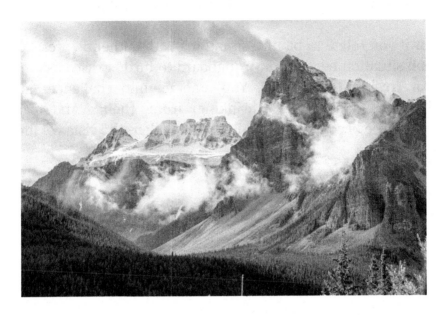

Beyond the habits and patterns of ordinary mind is another, more fundamental level of consciousness. This level of consciousness has no agenda or goal. It has nothing to prove, nothing to accomplish. It is self-sufficient and content. At this level there's no insecurity. There are no games to be played.

But this level of consciousness is not just mental blankness or stupidity. It's fundamentally aware, curious, open, and radiant. It is very sharp and clear. Like a crystal ball, it reflects everything. It is completely transparent, without any spots to obscure it. It is authentic presence.

Authentic presence is always there, somewhere in the background. Normally we don't see it. It's not that it's such a big secret or that we have to go digging deep into ourselves to find it. We're just facing the wrong direction.

Authentic presence is not just a personal experience, however, but a way of living your life. So it has both an inner and an outer side.

It is *authentic* because it is beyond the manipulations, games, stories, and stale emotional patterns of our ego. At the same time, when you *live* authentic presence, you are generous to others – generous with your very being. This is radical openness and honesty, which is another dimension of authenticity.

It is *presence* because it dwells within you already. It's already there; it's present. And you find it when you stay within the present moment. When you make it a part of your life, you are always present within life's situations, and you are genuinely present and available in your relationships with others.

Authentic presence is not just the opposite mode to ego. It's not like ego and authenticity are two opposing forces at war with each other. Rather, authentic presence is the very condition of ego in the first place. Ego can only take place because authentic presence is already there in the background.

This sounds like a paradox. How can authentic presence be at once the condition of ego as well as an alternative to it?

It's all a matter of how you place your awareness. Normally, we go through life on autopilot. We have our default ways of doing things and working with things. Because it's just too difficult, we don't often stray from this automatic mode. That requires a lot of sustained, conscious effort. Besides, it takes us out of our comfort zone. We've *evolved* our habits, defense mechanisms, and ego strategies for a reason. We've secreted a dense layer of ego around ourselves to protect ourselves from irritation and discomfort.

That's because our awareness is caught up in the logic of ego. There is me – and then there is the other. The other could be either a boon or a threat. Or it could just be uninteresting, something of no particular consequence to *me*. Our awareness is into figuring out the people, objects, and situations we encounter. Should we try to possess them – to hold on to them and make them our own? Or repel them, ward them off, fight them? Or can we just safely ignore them?

Even when we are in this agenda-driven mode, there is some spark of intelligence going on. It's not a condition of total darkness. There is some light shining through the murk, but its image is distorted, like a funhouse mirror. That spark of intelligence, that dim light, is the reflection of the authentic presence which always resides in the background, waiting to be discovered.

When we turn our awareness in its direction, the clouds begin to part, the fog begins to lift. Then the light becomes brighter and sharper. There is a greater sense of clarity. Inwardly, we have clarity and a sense of freshness and openness. Outwardly, engaged with the world, we feel curious and resourceful. That is, we not only have a sense that each new situation is a further opportunity for discovery – but we also have confidence in ourselves. We have confidence that opening ourselves up to experience and to other people is not going to destroy us. And we feel rich and resourceful. We feel that we have many inner resources for relating with our lives. The logic of "self" and "other" becomes transparent to us. We begin to get the sense that these are just patterns of thought rather than the reality of things.

When the concepts of "self" and "other" start to fade away, we're easing into the experience of nonduality. "Nonduality" and "nondualism" are among the most abused words in the vocabulary of spirituality. Nondualism could easily be turned into a sophisticated philosophical system — and many have done just that. It doesn't help that it's so abstract.

But we don't need to construct a new system of thought. We don't have to make it so complicated. In fact, in practice, we should be aiming to *uncomplicate* things. That means disassembling the dualistic thought process.

Dualistic thought begins with self and other, I and not-I. This duality justifies the mechanical, agenda-driven action of ego. And that action in turn keeps churning out more and more dualistic thoughts. It's a vicious cycle, a feedback mechanism.

When you see someone coming, you quickly assess whether they're an enemy or friend. Is this person coming to harm me or help me? And based on how you answer that, then you determine how you'll act to that person — friendly or hostile. The whole engine of duality – friend versus enemy, good versus bad, pleasant or unpleasant, approach or retreat – runs on the fuel of self and other. That's ego's whole game.

To keep the narrative intact, ego will engage in every kind of manipulation and self-deception. It's like a politician trying to keep up the narrative of their campaign.

Did you ever see *House of Cards?* Ego is like a little Frank Underwood running around, trying to move all the pieces here and there. It's all about managing perceptions, making sure every part of the story is airtight so the light of truth can't show through the cracks. If we let too much light in, it might blow the lid off the whole thing. Then we might see how dirty and grubby our little cave is. We're quite afraid of seeing that, because at least it's *our* cave, and the world out there is too unpredictable and scary.

But we could let that all fall away. We just let it go, drop it like a dirty set of clothes and step out into the nakedness of the authentic state.

The authentic state is *non*dual because the dualistic thoughts that dominate our ego-driven mode simply don't exist in that space. Dualistic thought is all about creating points of reference, comparing this to that and making sure this is pinned down and that is pigeonholed, and so on.

But when you're dwelling in authentic presence, there is no reference point. There's no self or other to hang your hat on.

I don't want to overly theorize about it. There's no reason to bury this authentic state in abstractions and speculations. How could the sky itself be carved into some definite shape? Though we do need some sort of theory of ego, that's just to untangle ego's knotted web of concepts. As for the authentic presence, it has to be experienced to be understood. That begins with getting a glimpse. And the way to do that is through the practice of meditation.

Chapter 3. Sitting

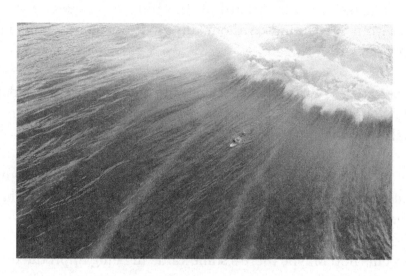

Resting

The word "meditation" is very intimidating. It sounds like there's something to do, and you're not quite sure what it is or how to do it. Whatever it is, it sounds like a chore.

Maybe there's some better word for it, like "resting." That we could relate to. We all rest sometimes. We sleep, watch a movie we like, go for a walk, sit outside somewhere and enjoy the scenery, listen to some good music. So we all know what it's like to relax and enjoy ourselves, and we don't have to be told how to do it. It's not like there are many steps involved.

Meditation doesn't have to be practiced like some austere discipline. It's not a stern exercise regimen that you force yourself through, or a boot camp where a drill sergeant is screaming down at you as you do pushups. It's not about giving yourself a headache or backache trying to sit perfectly still and straight. It's not about about forcing your mind to concentrate on something.

It's a chance to give yourself a break. Give your ego a break. Don't make it work so hard all the time. Sometimes just sit with your own mind, without any plan or agenda, and just hang out with yourself.

That's a very rewarding experience in itself, because we seldom allow ourselves such a luxury. Just sit down without a plan or goal? Who has time for that? It sounds very unproductive.

But whoever said we have to be productive all the time? Where is that written down? Even if it's written down somewhere, so what? Were we born on this earth to be productive and then die?

It seems not. Maybe there's some value in being unproductive.

If you think I'm wrong about that, then at least give it a try. Prove me wrong rather than just writing me off. If you've really tried *resting* or meditation, then you can say with authority, "Meditation is a waste of time."

Even if you like what I'm saying, then *still* try to prove me wrong. If you just took my word for it, you'd be pretty gullible. So in either case, you should try it out for yourself just to find out what all the fuss is about. Then you will really know the value of being unproductive.

Getting to Know Yourself

There are no shortcuts here. You have to sit down with your mind. You have to spend a lot of time with your mind in meditation. Let's dispel some common misconceptions. Meditation is not some mystical path for achieving union with God. It's not a system of therapy that's meant to fix whatever is troubling you – anxiety, depression, stress, whatever.

24

(Although it can and will make you feel better, if you stick with it. But that's not the point.)

Meditation is best approached without such fixed ideas or goals in mind. It's best to approach it with a sense of curiosity. Yes, something *will* come of meditating – but what will that be? It remains to be discovered. Not knowing can bring inspiration. It can motivate you to discover for yourself.

When you're getting to know a person, if you really are getting to know them, you don't have fixed expectations about who they are and what they are like. Meditation is just like that. It's a process of getting to know yourself. So you have to be ready to drop your ideas about what you'll find. You have to be open to the possibility that there might be some surprises. You don't quite know what to expect, but still you can have some sense of expectation.

To get to know yourself, you have to carve out time for yourself. That's just a matter of respect and kindness. If you respect someone and want to be kind to them, you will make time for them. If you respect yourself and want to be kind to yourself, you'll make time for yourself. Even if you have a very busy schedule, somehow you'll figure out a way to give five to ten minutes, at least, to yourself.

You might be thinking that it sounds strange to talk about getting to know yourself. How can you not know yourself? My only response is to give it a shot. You'll be surprised about how much you didn't know and how much there is to discover.

Maybe you have some fixed ideas about yourself. These are ego's stories that it tells itself. Do you think that you're bad? You might discover that you're good. Do you think you're good? You might discover your dark side – the selfish and hurtful things that you do. The point is not to shy away from such discoveries, good or bad. You have to be willing to sit with yourself and see your own mind plainly. That's why meditation is an expression of courage and compassion. You have the courage to look into yourself without knowing in advance what you will find. You have the compassion to face it all without judgment, but empathy.

How to Sit

At this point we have to start talking in very practical terms. We have to talk about technique. We've now got a sense of where we are and where we'd like to be. If you're still with me, then you're probably wanting to break out of the stale habitual patterns of ego and find a new way of relating to your world.

That all starts with just finding some time in the day to sit on your butt and look at your mind. Some caveats apply. First, if you're going to do it properly, you need to make it a daily practice. It can't just be a sometime thing. Second, however much time you give to yourself, you can't let it be violated. Five minutes or two hours, it doesn't matter. Unless a fire breaks out, you don't leave your cushion.

That brings us to equipment. The only equipment you'll really need is a cushion that you can sit comfortably on for however long you choose to meditate. It needs to be high enough that your legs are at the optimal angle – sloping slightly from hips to knees, which are on the ground. That allows your spine to stay straight. It needs to be firm enough to support your spine. It also needs to be soft enough that you don't feel sore from sitting on it. There are many cushions available on the market that are made just for meditation, so it shouldn't be hard to find one.

The best position is cross-legged on the floor, preferably on the carpet to go easy on your knees and ankles. But if you have some pain in your back or legs that prevents you from sitting that way, then you can also sit in a chair. The key point is that your spine should be held straight. Don't hold it too stiffly or there will be tension and pain. But in a relaxed matter, keep it straight for as long as you sit. This straight position helps you to keep your awareness steady. Imagine that your spine is a stack of coins. It can't lean too far either forward or backward without toppling over. Or imagine that there's a string tied to the crown of your head, and it's gently pulling you from above. That will help you get a feel for the right position.

When you sit down, you should have a sense of dignity. The meditation cushion is your throne, and you are like a king or queen. What you are doing is not awkward or embarrassing at all, but very dignified. It's the most dignified, majestic thing you could do – sitting with courage and grace and looking at your mind.

When you first sit down, take at least a few moments to become aware of your body. Double check to see if your posture is good. Feel the weight of your body on the cushion beneath you. Feel your knees against the floor. Notice if your body is feeling cool or hot. Notice if there is any muscle tension in your body. If there is, try to relax those muscles. If not, just feel the already relaxed state of your body. If you want, you can concentrate your awareness on an imaginary point underground, some two or three meters beneath you. That will help to ground you and get you out of your head. It will bring your awareness into your body and into the present moment.

The usual point of departure for meditation is to practice mindfulness of the breath. And for a beginner, the easiest way to do that is to count the breath. You don't have to alter the breath or make it long or short. Just leave it as it is naturally. When you breathe in, *One*. When you breathe out, *Two*. Count up to ten, then start over from the beginning.

At first, counting can be your entire meditation practice. With time, this technique will come to seem too heavy-handed. Then you can just rest your attention on the sensation of the breath as it goes in and out of your nostrils. Just feel what the breath is like – whether it's cool or hot, long or short, heavy or light.

The breath is an ideal object for meditation because, while it's physical and definite, it's also subtle and light. It also tunes your mind to the rhythms of the body and brings body and mind together in the present moment. When you're meditating on the breath, don't try to force your awareness into an overbearing concentration. At the same time, don't just let your mind go straying around wherever it wants. You want to have some discipline, but not a heavy, brutal discipline. Just rest your attention lightly on the breath. This will take some practice, but with time, you'll get the hang of it.

When your mind gets distracted and wanders off, just gently bring your attention back to the breath. If you were counting, start again from *One*. There's no need to feel bad that you got distracted. Whatever thoughts come up, you don't have to get involved with them. They are not good or bad. They're just thoughts, passing thoughts. They come and go, no big deal. Just bring your attention back to the breath.

If your posture slips and you're leaning back or forward, or if you're slouching, then you will get distracted or sleepy. So when you catch yourself in distraction, briefly check your posture and make any adjustments. If you feel pain and need to move a bit, go ahead and do that. But small adjustments are better than large adjustments. If you move around a lot, it will disturb the balance of your mind and make your attention more restless.

Looking at Your Mind

So far we've only talked about the breath. As you get more and more familiar with the practice, your attention will become more and more subtle and stable. It will not be moved to distraction so easily, but simply rest on the breath for long periods of time without wavering. You will come to know the flavor of a very refined and subtle level of attention that you didn't have before.

It may take a lot of time practicing meditation to achieve this level of attention, or you might achieve it very quickly. The point is, when you do find that your attention is very focused and light, you can let it go. You no longer have to try to direct it at the breath, but you can just rest in a general awareness of the present moment. You might find that this awareness is incredibly peaceful, clear, and pleasant. At this point, you don't have to direct your attention at anything in particular. You don't need to rely on an object of meditation. But if thoughts arise, you can just watch them come up. If a feeling occurs, you can just observe it and feel its qualities.

The point of this is to practice looking at your mind. It's much easier to do this if your mind is very calm and clear. It's like looking through a pool of water. If the water is agitated, then the mud will be disturbed from the bottom of the pool. It will become murky and dark. When you leave the water alone, its movements and ripples eventually subside. The mud settles to the bottom. Then you can see through the water as clearly as you could through a window. It becomes completely transparent.

We're trying to make our mind transparent so that we can see it clearly. At the same time, we don't reject anything that comes up or try to force it down. We simply let it be, and it comes to rest on its own. Don't try to put a stop to the ripples and waves on the surface of the mind – just watch them and let them subside on their own.

We're also allowing for the possibility for something remarkable to happen. If you can calm your mind down to this point, so that it becomes very clear and steady, then you might have a sudden experience of all thought and grasping falling away. It's as if the world suddenly opened up around you and became very sharp and vivid. You yourself become transparent or insubstantial, as if someone could throw a stone at you and it would just go right through you. It's like a fresh wind just blew through you, or like you were crawling through a tunnel, but suddenly you're standing in a great, open meadow, with green grass all around you and the sun shining in the blue sky above you. The taste of this experience is incredibly refreshing and pure.

This is the experience of authentic presence. It might last for only the briefest moment. But in that moment, all the habits, grasping, patterns, and agendas of ego just fall away. What is left is just pure awareness.

That is what *you* are, fundamentally, beneath all your thoughts and emotions. That is what you are, beyond all the flotsam and jetsam of the ordinary mind. At the same time, it's not *you*, because there's no sense of "I" or "me" to hold on to.

This experience can't be prolonged or had by trying to hold on to it. Think of holding a wet bar of soap. If you tighten your grip, it will just slip away from you. But if you let it rest loosely in your palm, it will stay there.

Just letting it rest takes a lot of practice, actually. The tendency to grasp tightly is such a deeply engrained habit of the mind. And for most of us, letting go and letting be are not really our strong suit. But with time, you will have more glimpses of this state. They will become longer and more familiar. You will be able to touch on it at will. And that's when you'll be able to bring it into your daily life.

Distractions and Experiences

All kinds of thoughts and feelings come up in meditation. These shouldn't be regarded as a problem. When you first start meditating, it will be very easy for mental excitation to sweep you up in its current, or to sink into a dull or sleepy state. With time, you will start to recognize such distractions as soon as they're happening.

Sometimes you are sitting, minding the breath, and then a few minutes later you realize that your mind wandered off to the beach, or to how you haven't gotten around to doing your taxes, or to some piece of gossip you heard. There's no need to punish yourself or to feel bad about your mind slipping off like that. Distractions are a natural part of the process. As long as you're committing time each day to sitting down with yourself, you're doing well. Simply bring your mind back and rest it again.

Another thing that might happen is that curious experiences arise. You might have visions or dreamlike imagery. Maybe you suddenly feel overwhelmed with a sense of bliss – or fear.

Or you might have distorted perceptions, such as some part of your body becoming very large or small. All sorts of strange experiences can arise.

It's best to ignore such experiences. But if they're too powerful, they can become a hangup for your practice. You might be either too attached or too disturbed, depending on the experience. In such cases it's best to stop your meditation session and to stand up and go wash the dishes or something. If you get very attached to, say, an experience of bliss, then every time you sit down, you'll try to recreate that experience. When you fail, you'll get discouraged with meditation and might even give it up altogether. Or if you have a very disturbing experience, that could make you afraid to sit down on the cushion. So if an experience comes up that's too extreme, it's best just to leave the cushion and find something else to do. Then, the next day, sit down again and continue your practice.

Boredom

Normally when we feel bored, we get very restless and immediately search for some entertainment to fill the gap and relieve the feeling of boredom. Boredom comes from a lack of stimulation, which means you get too close to your own thoughts and your own mind. And that becomes very uncomfortable. So we try to push the mind farther away by creating some external entertainment.

I'm bored, let's watch a movie. That's a very innocent way to handle boredom. But sometimes we do something reckless or harmful just to relieve that feeling. There's no end to the kind of mischief we can get up to because of boredom.

32

When you're meditating, boredom gets very irritating, because you can't do anything about it. You feel an itch, but you have to keep the discipline of not scratching it. But your mind stays on the itch. The itch becomes bigger and bigger until it fills your mind completely. You can't think about anything else except how that itch is screaming out to be scratched.

Meditation doesn't give you an outlet for boredom. It doesn't allow you to entertain yourself or find relief. Sure, you can stand up from your seat and go to the mall or turn on the TV. But then you're not meditating anymore. You *were* meditating, then you dropped it and did something else.

So boredom can really leave you squirming where you sit. Sometimes you find yourself like that, physically moving or fidgeting because the boredom becomes so uncomfortable.

Meditation has many, many moments of boredom. You're bored because you're alone with your mind, and there's nothing you can use to distract yourself from that. You can't escape, which drives you crazy. You're there on the spot, and boredom is poking you.

You have to just deal with whatever is there. All of your thoughts, good or bad, pleasant or painful, ordinary, stupid, clever, creative, humdrum, exciting, twisted, violent, weird, jealous, obsessive — whatever is there, you have to stay with it, because that's the practice.

It turns out what's boring you is your own dualistic thoughts. They are so stale and old, and you have had them for so long, that you experience them as a tremendous drag. You don't really know how to stop this self-perpetuating ego machine once you've turned it on, but you want to do anything but spend more time with it.

Ego's games are so boring, so repetitive, not subtle or clever or amusing at all. So you involve yourself in all kinds of entertainment to escape them.

In meditation, there's no direction to go but deeper *into* the boredom. The more you go into it, the less you feel that you need some relief. You become less and less desperate to do something to get rid of boredom. The boredom itself begins to settle down.
At that point, it's hard to say if it's even boredom anymore. If boredom is some kind of restless feeling, then it's no longer that. It's just the quiet feeling of being where you are and nowhere else. Your mind becomes very settled. You're totally just into the practice of hanging out with yourself, getting to know your own mind.

Nothing seems boring because every thought and emotion that arises is vivid and unique, at the same time as being one with the totality of your experience. It feels very relaxed and spacious. You learn to relax into the spaces in your mental chatter, when things become silent, and it's not so uncomfortable for you anymore.

Emotions

Emotions are very powerful. They have the power to move us to action with huge consequences.

Anger, for example, can destroy friendships, relationships, and even lives. Love can bring people together and cause two people to make life-altering choices. Sadness can leave you brooding alone in your home, neglecting your life.

When emotions arise in meditation, they are disturbing because they have such tremendous energy. Somehow, all that energy pushing you in one direction or another makes the simple discipline of sitting down very difficult to keep.

Boredom can make you squirm or fall asleep. But emotions come at you with such force and urgency that sitting still becomes excruciating. You might be all the way up from your cushion before you even realize you lost your meditation.

There is a school of thought that says you should just surrender to your emotions. You should let them take over and play out on their own. This school of thought says that it's healthy to act out your anger, for example. Just let its violent force play out through your actions. Do you feel frustrated? Just lash out. It's cathartic.

This way of handling emotions has nothing to do with meditation or authentic presence. The word for it is *selfishness*. Contrary to received wisdom, it's not healthy, but extremely destructive.

Yes, in meditation, we don't try to kill our emotions. We don't try to perform an amputation to remove the emotional part of ourselves. But that doesn't mean we get completely swept up in their current, either.

On the other hand, there is a temptation, especially if the emotion is very powerful, to suppress it or talk yourself out of it. But this is a bad strategy.

Actually, it's dead awful, for a few reasons. For one, suppressing the emotion doesn't get rid of it. It just pushes it below the surface.

It makes you feel anxious and restless. You're not quite sure what's wrong, because you already suppressed the emotion. It's somewhere down there, below the threshold, eating at you. You can feel it chewing at you from the inside, but you don't know what it is.

But the real problem with suppressing emotions is that you lose a chance to look at them directly. You lose the chance to relate to them with genuineness and a willingness to understand their nature. And so you miss out on the opportunity to go deeper into authenticity.

Emotions seem threatening because they are not just forceful, but they seem very solid and real. But if we look at them closely, we find out that what used to seem solid just falls apart.

Look at emotions closely. What are they, really? What are they made of? Do they have any definite shape or texture?

It turns out they're very fluid and changing. They consist of a feeling in the body, and over that feeling is a layer of discursive thought.

Anger might feel like a flush of heat in the face, a tension in the limbs, clenched fists. On top of that is a story that you tell yourself. *He insulted me, hurt me. I have to stand up for myself and show that I won't be taken advantage of.*

So you don't just watch the movie, so to speak. You also get the director's commentary, which is constantly running and saying, *This means X, Y, Z,* and so on. So emotions are made up of the raw energy of the emotion, plus that heavy layer of interpretation.

The way to relate to emotions from a standpoint of authentic presence is just to drop the interpretation. Let the director's commentary go. Let yourself feel the energy. Just allow yourself to feel it fully. Feel its texture, experience its color and vividness.

With practice, you'll discover that often, the energy of feeling is a kind of communication. Maybe it's alerting you to the fact that something is wrong within yourself or your environment. Maybe it's calling your attention to some possibility. The only sure thing is that you're going to miss the plot if the director's commentary is on.

There's no guidebook to this. I can tell you how to ride a horse. I can give you every technical detail about how it's done. But there will be something left over, something I can't tell you. That you can only learn from getting on top of the horse and riding it yourself. Then you will become familiar with the horse, with all its habits and moods. And with a lot of experience, you'll become an expert rider.

Insight

At this point it might be helpful to introduce a kind of Buddhist meditation, which is called *insight meditation*. The point of doing insight meditation is not to turn you into a Buddhist. You don't have to accept any of the dogmas or trappings of Buddhism.

But the method is very useful for loosening your sense of identification with your body, thoughts, and emotions. These identifications are the basis of ego. Ego is based on the concept *I am* this, *and* that *is other than me.*

If you look at your experience, you'll find that all of it is made up of physical and mental elements. There are sensations of sight, smell, hearing, taste, and touch. Then there are thoughts, memories, emotions, daydreams, feelings, and so on.

If you're a skeptical type and don't believe that the physical and mental are separate things, that's fine. For the purposes of this meditation, you don't have to believe that. The point is that there are experiences that have a more physical flavor and experiences that have a more mental flavor.

For example, the taste of salt has a definitely physical flavor. It immediately presses itself on our senses. The quality of a thought, however, is not physically definite at all. It seems to exist in some abstract space. Whether or not that's really the case is beside the point. We *experience* it that way, and that's enough for this exercise.

So if we divide up experience, we have roughly the physical and mental. Physical experiences include sensations like the vividness of a bright blue or the texture of cotton. Mental experiences include thoughts, feelings, memories, emotions, and so on.

Once your attention is very refined and stable through the practice of meditation we described earlier, then you can point it towards the physical and mental elements of your experience and analyze them.

So, let's say, while you're in meditation a cold breeze touches your skin and you get goosebumps. You then analyze this experience, asking yourself, "Is this experience me? Am I this experience? Is it mine?"

You keep going like this, looking at every experience you have and trying to find the *self*. We all believe that we have a self, or are a self. That's the whole idea of ego in the first place. So if there's a self, it must be somewhere within our experience. So we look at everything that comes up in our experience and scrutinize it to see if it's the self we're looking for.

If you look at all your physical sensations and decide that the self is not the body, then it's time to look at everything that comes up in the mind. Start with your feelings – your sense that any given experience is pleasant or unpleasant, good or bad. Scrutinize these and look for the ego.

If you don't find it there, look at your emotions. Then consider your thoughts. Then consider the consciousness that is thinking the thoughts.

If you think you've found the self somewhere, then look more closely. Say you think you found the self, and it's the consciousness that's doing the thinking. Consider this consciousness in more detail. Does it change, or does it stay the same? If it changes, is it the same consciousness from moment to moment, or is something new coming into being? If it's not the same, can it really be the self?

Because the self would have to be the same over a long period of time in order to really be "you." Otherwise you are not the same person you were yesterday.

Is there just one consciousness happening at a time, or are there several? Or do you switch back and forth between the difference consciousnesses? Is consciousness a steady and continuous thing, or does it flicker in and out? What happens to it when you go to sleep? Do "you" stop existing? Where is consciousness, exactly? Is it in your head or your chest? What does it feel like?

These are not just abstract or philosophical questions. They are about your own experience, how you approach it.

Through this exercise, you really look at experience closely and discover that it's really just a stream of events. The only constant is that the pace of change never slackens, even when you're relaxed and not much is going on around you. Even in those conditions, there is a constant flux, and endless stream of sensations, thoughts, emotions, and so on.

So where is the self in all this? If you're clever, you've figured out that the point of this search is to come up empty handed. Having searched all through your own experience, you find there are no more candidates for "self" left. This will help loosen your identity with ego and bring you closer into authentic presence.

Chapter 4. Living

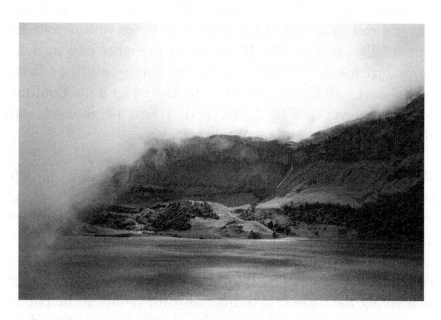

Touching on Authentic Presence

Authentic presence is not just something that you practice on the meditation cushion. Meditation is simply the best way to discover it within yourself. It's time-tested – tried and true. For thousands of years, spiritual seekers have been practicing meditation, and millions of them have found the authentic presence within themselves in just this way.

But it's not enough just to sit on your butt and let your mental manipulations drop. You actually have to get off the cushion at some point and live your life. And when you do, you can either go back to the old, ego-driven habits, or you can bring your newfound sense of peace and clarity into life.

There are many common, humdrum activities of life that are perfect opportunities for bringing the quality of authentic awareness into what you're doing. Throughout the day, you can bring authentic presence into what you're doing by simply touching on it. The glimpses that you experience in meditation you can call to mind. Simply find that space within yourself, that totally open quality that lets all thoughts and agendas drop. Just touch on it for a moment. Then – and this is the crucial part – don't try to hold on to it. Just let it go. Continue doing whatever you're doing, and it will be infused with authentic presence quite naturally.

This technique is so easy and useful because you don't have to force anything. You simply bring authentic presence into your living situations and let it do its work naturally. With practice, that kind of awareness will become easy and natural.

To start with, you can practice this in neutral situations, such as washing the dishes, cleaning the yard, watering the plants, fixing a sandwich, washing your hands. These situations don't present any special challenges, but they can be boring. We usually just perform such tasks automatically while our minds are elsewhere. In the practice of authentic presence, we don't want to just go through the motions. That's too mechanical, too lifeless.

When you bring authentic presence into your daily activities, you feel them and experience them properly. Doing the dishes is such a simple yet such an important task. They have to get clean. There's something very direct and good about it. The dish is dirty. You use soap and hot water to make it clean. There's a problem and a solution, and a direct action that gets it done without any fuss.

In time you should bring this technique into your dealings with other people. When you're talking to them, you can just touch on the experience of authentic presence – then let it go.

It will transform the way you relate to people. You will soften up, become more open. Because you are being more genuine, the way they relate to you will also change. People will notice the changes in you and remark on them. They might say that you have become very relaxed, or easygoing. Or they might even say you seem sad – just because you're calm and they don't know how to interpret that! You don't have to take it too seriously. It's just a reminder that others notice the changes that you're experiencing within yourself.

Living Ethically

There's no blueprint or formula for living with authentic presence. Formulas and blueprints are just another kind of manipulation, another strategy. The only agenda in authentic presence is to have no agenda. Instead, you relate to living situations as they occur. If you are placing your mind in the space of authentic presence, then your actions will simply be a natural extension of that. Quite naturally, you will be open and honest with others. Because you won't be trying to push your agenda, you'll actually be able to *hear* them and *see* them.

There is an ethical dimension to living a spiritual life. If you are practicing "spirituality" but not living ethically, then you're full of crap. You're kidding yourself. There's nothing genuine about such spirituality.

Consumer-oriented, pop-culture mindfulness has been marketed very effectively to the public. Critics call this consumer-friendly version of spirituality "McMindfulness." It's an apt name. The contemporary mindfulness brand being sold to the public has a nice taste. It's a pleasant vacation from the stresses of life. But it lacks depth. It lacks a moral dimension.

Truth be told, that moral dimension is the hardest part to get right. Our culture and psychology tell us it's all about our happiness, our self-expression, self-determination, protecting our rights, cultivating a strong sense of self. The constant refrain is *me, me, me*.

That's very good advice for living in a conventional way that doesn't contradict the priorities of the world. By following this advice, we could become master deceivers, master manipulators of ourselves and others. We could convince ourselves that we've built a very strong sense of self and have all this self-confidence. We could even keep that up for a long time.

But it would be based on a lie. Sooner or later, we'd be confronted with the fact that self-esteem and self-confidence are all propped up by external reference points. We can write a very good resume or C.V., but it turns out that our credentials are all bullshit. What happens when we're deprived of our credentials? Then we find out how weak our sense of self was all along.

As we've already seen, the path of authentic presence is not about cultivating a robust ego. It's about undoing the web of self-deception which is ego's modus operandi. What's left over is indestructible, because it doesn't rely on crutches or a good story. It just is, like the sky. Like space, it's the basic condition that makes everything possible and the place where everything occurs.

There was nothing to protect to begin with, so the whole exercise of ego was a big joke. Therefore we can surrender all of the credentials, surrender this big ego, and be genuine to ourselves and others. Loosen our grip and expose our raw hearts to the world. That what's meant by the moral dimension of authentic presence.

From a genuinely spiritual standpoint, ethics begins with the understanding that every person has fundamental value. Just as you have your own inner world, just as you contain a universe within yourself, so does each person you encounter in your life. They all have their hopes and dreams, their fears, resentments, memories, likes and dislikes. They have their moments of wonder. They have people who love them and people whom they love. They have a longing for something more, for something truer and better than the small world ego has made for them. And they have, within themselves, the clarity and openness of authentic presence, whether they recognize it or not. So treat them that way.

That is another way of stating the Golden Rule: Treat others as you want them to treat you. The Golden Rule contains the recognition that others are just like us, and our behavior should reflect that. If you act like you're more important than others, then you're not just being selfish. You're making an error of belief. It's as if you were on one side of the street, and a man stood next to you. On the opposite side of the street stood another man. The man closer to you appears taller, to your vision. And just because of that, you think that the man who is close to you is actually large, and the one who's far away is actually small.

People are not more or less important, more or less valuable, just because they are close to us or distant from us. Near to us or not, everyone is valuable. Just like you, they want to be happy. They don't want to suffer.

So to live with authentic presence, on an ethical level, means at the very least not hurting anybody. Abandon any action that harms others. That includes abuse both verbal and physical, using people for selfish ends, deception, cheating, stealing, and so on. If you can, help people who are in need. But if you can't do that, at least don't hurt them.

Authentic Presence in the Workplace

A huge percentage of our life is spent working, and if we don't bring authentic presence into the workplace, we're missing a tremendous opportunity to open ourselves up to new ways of relating to our work. Work is a very honest and direct way of relating to the world. It's very simple. You need money to live. You need to work to make money. There are no shortcuts here. Sure, it's possible to make easy money in a number of ways, some of them dishonest. But doing that is just another way of trying to manipulate things to your advantage. That will only take you farther away from authentic presence.

Other kinds of work might be harmful to others. One example is selling weapons. Another is selling products that are harmful to people's health – food that contains poisonous chemicals, for example. You don't have to be obsessed about organic food, if that's not your thing. The idea is just to examine your livelihood and be honest about whether it helps people or harms them. If it harms them, it's best to find another line of work.

Living ethically is not meant to be a punishment or a burden. It's not about laying a guilt trip on anyone. But there are some kinds of action that bring you closer to authentic presence, and some kinds that take you farther away. The actions that bring you closer are the ones that are direct, honest, and harmless. And practicing this in the work that you do is an excellent way to deepen your experience of authenticity in your life.

There are also many challenges that come up in the way you relate to people in your workplace. The workplace is filled with many people, each with their own dreams, desires, ambitions, neuroses, and hang-ups. A lot of friction happens. It's not uncommon for people to butt heads when their goals are incompatible.

It's not always possible to completely relinquish your agenda at work. We all have many responsibilities in life, after all, so we can't just give in to others when that means neglecting our responsibilities. But at least, when a conflict arises, you can try to understand the other side. Open up and really listen to what the other person is saying to you, instead of planning how to get back at them or get around them. Try to understand their point of view, why it's important to them, how they feel, why they are behaving the way they are.

Instead of seeing how the other person advances or impedes your agenda, you could see them with the freshness of authentic presence. Here is a person, a fellow human being. What makes them tick? What is their story? Why do they do the things they do? You could regard the people in your life with curiosity. If you see them this way, it's much more natural to treat people as ends in themselves, rather than as a means to your ends.

You'd be surprised how many conflicts can be resolved this way. Often you can reach a solution that accommodates every party, or at least meet them in the middle with a compromise.

Here, as elsewhere, we can practice briefly touching on authentic presence and letting it suffuse our activities. As we go about our work, and when we are engaging with others in the workplace, it's important to return again and again to our center so we can bring its peaceful and creative energy into our work life.

Nowhere in our lives do we find ourselves in more intimate or vulnerable situations than we do in our personal relationships – including with family members, but most especially with a spouse or partner. The kitchen is a great metaphor for this. It's a domestic space, where we produce sustenance for our bodies – very basic, but very important. That's like our personal relationships. Because we're always in the same kitchen, so to speak, bumping against each other, relationships generate a lot of friction. We come to know each other inside and out – not just likes, dislikes, opinions, and habits, but each other's most personal thoughts, feelings, insecurities, doubts, hopes, fears, dreams, and fantasies.

This leaves us open to being used and hurt by others. Just as importantly, if we're not careful, we might find ourselves unconsciously using and hurting the ones we love. But our personal relationships also offer unsurpassed opportunities to get to know ourselves and others. The friction of a relationship contains tremendous energy. Because it is so close, so personal, that friction actually generates sparks that can ignite our practice of authentic presence.

In spite – or maybe because – of the intensity of the situations that arise in relationships, it is even more important to bring mindfulness and openness into the picture. As before, we can practice the technique of touching on authentic presence. But we need to bring extra care and attentiveness into how we relate to those close to us, because our situation is so intimate and so sensitive.

Authentic presence in the context of relationships means not just trying to push your agenda. It means not just getting pulled into a tug-of-war with those who you're close to. Sometimes, surrendering ego's agenda in a relationship is a way to spur on growth and bring you closer to another. It can bring them also to drop their defenses. It can melt through the ice that sometimes forms in a relationship in which each party has hardened their position.

The open, aware, sharp, penetrating, clear, compassionate, and accommodating quality of authentic presence that you've cultivated through the practice of meditation can be brought into your relationships. When there are problems or arguments, it can open the way to creative solutions. If you show empathy to your partner or family member, they are more likely to drop their agenda and show empathy to you.

Too often relationships are based on the need to control the other person. We feel that we need them. That makes us vulnerable. If they left us or did not return our love, where would we be? So we try to control them or possess them to remove the threat of that possibility. We might be clinging to someone who wants to leave. Or we might be better off if we left our partner, but we hold on to them out of fear.

If we're dwelling in authentic presence, there's nothing to fear, nothing to hold on to. We don't have to try to control others or maintain control of our situation. We can let them be. Ironically, this approach is more likely to help a relationship last. If the relationship has a good foundation with two people who are willing to give of themselves and understand each other, then relinquishing the need to secure the relationship gives it some breathing room. It allows it to thrive.

Chapter 5. Problems

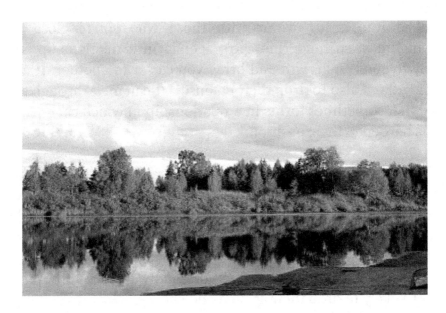

Giving Up Control

Remember how I said that insecurity is like a seed, and it finds rich soil in the mind? The soil of the mind is authentic presence. It is the ground itself. Without this soil, nothing can grow – good or bad. The soil itself doesn't care whether a garden is grown on it or it gets taken over by weeds. On that question it's neutral. The nature of soil is just to be rich, fertile, and nurturing. It accommodates any kind of life.

Likewise, authentic presence can accommodate any kind of thought, feeling, or situation. Because it has nothing to defend or prove, it doesn't have to try to change anything. It can just let things be without trying to manipulate them.

That might sound paradoxical. If authentic presence doesn't try to change negativity, then what is so great about it? How can it actually make our lives better?

But that is precisely what is so good about it. It's the absence of games and manipulations. It's just *authentic,* natural, and easy. In practice, when you're living with authentic presence, then whenever ego games come up, they just kind of wear themselves out and settle down on their own accord. Authentic presence doesn't try to lay hold of ego and say, "Now, calm down!" It just opens a window onto ego's room and waits for it to relax, stop defending itself, and come outside. On this level, nothing has to be done.

In *Zen Mind, Beginner's Mind,* Sunryu Suzuki Roshi gives a wonderful example of how we try to control things. We try to control people as well as our own minds, but the result is that we lose control of them. They rebel against our pushing an agenda on them. Suzuki Roshi says that the best way to control a cow is not to try to force your will on it, but to give it a big grassy meadow. The cow will wander around, eat some grass, and finally relax and come to rest by itself. That is how you "control" a cow.

So it is with our own thoughts. When we're abiding in authentic presence, we have no agenda. We just give our thoughts and emotions, our games and manipulations, a big open space in which to do their thing. After some time, they run out of steam and come to relax on their own. But if we try to control them, we only end up feeding more energy into the egosystem.

Negativity Is Not Negative

In truth, we can't control our thoughts or feelings. We can only create the right conditions for happy thoughts and feelings to thrive. But without the feedback of negativity, we're deprived of a valuable source of information. "Negativity" is not always negative. It often gives us a timely message that something is wrong. Something needs to be attended to.

Let's not kid ourselves. Happiness is not a matter of telling yourself, "I am happy" or "I want to be happy." When you think about such "positive affirmations," they sound like a bad joke. The truth is that sometimes life knocks you to the ground. Or you just knock yourself to the ground. It doesn't matter, because whatever the case, when you hit the ground, it hurts. Life's knocks are painful.

Living life with authentic presence is not about rejecting the pain. It is not about finding a cure. Rather, it's about the recognition that nothing needed to be cured to begin with. But to get to that point, first you have to be spurred on by your pain. At the very least, there has to be some kind of dissatisfaction that drives you onto the path of authenticity. And it drives you because you can't bear it somehow.

So that's the paradox of this path: We are driven to it, awakened to our need for it, because we can't bear our pain, irritation, and longing. But the path itself is about learning to accommodate that same suffering and dissatisfaction within the larger field of authentic presence. That is what makes authentic presence so powerful. It's a state of being that accommodates everything. It embraces the full spectrum of life, good and bad.

When we are willing to embrace negativity, to work with it and invite it to our table, we allow communication to take place. The negativity itself becomes less painful. And because we no longer perceive it as a threat, it's able to impart its message to us.

But that's easier said than done. When powerful negative thoughts and emotions come up, it's so easy to get swept up in their current. It's much more difficult to find the presence of authentic awareness within ourselves, which opens us up and gives negativity the space it needs to settle down and give its message.

One technique that I find to be especially helpful is given by the meditation teacher Tara Brach. It's a simple process for recovering the state of authentic presence when turmoil comes along and allows for emotional healing to occur. She calls it R.A.I.N., which stands for *Recognition* of what's happening, *Allowing* life to be as it is, *Investigating* your state of mind with kindness, and *Non-identification* with the negative thoughts or emotions that are occurring.

1. The first stage, *recognition*, means that when a difficult emotional situation first turns up, you stop and take stock of what's happening right now. Pay attention to your emotional state. *Recognize* it. Ask yourself what is going on in your mind right now, and really look. Just look at your mind and see. How is your current state of mind? How's the weather in there, so to speak? Just check it out and see.

2. The next stage kind of comes along with the first. It means you *allow* things to be as they are. Don't try to change anything or fix it, or apply some kind of solution. Don't try to suppress your emotions or distract your mind with activity or entertainment. But whatever is there, let it be. Let it just hang out in its own space, through the ever-accommodating practice of authentic presence. It's not good or bad, per se. It just *is*, it's happening right now, and whatever is happening inside is okay. If it helps, you can tell yourself verbally, "I accept my emotions and will let them simply be in the state of authentic presence."

At this point you might already have reconnected with the experience of authentic presence. If that's the case, you can just rest your mind in that state. There's no need to apply further techniques. The R.A.I.N. process is meant to bring you back into the state of meditative openness, so mission accomplished.

3. But if that didn't do the trick, you can continue with *investigation* of your mental state. Ask yourself why you feel this way, what caused this emotion? Without putting any blame on anybody, try to understand what it is about this particular situation that sets off this particular emotion. What beliefs support or sustain your current emotional state? Where do you feel it in your body? What is the message this negative emotion is trying to communicate?

The point of this inquiry is to look at yourself with kindness. You don't need to point a finger at yourself or beat yourself. Just look at yourself with a sense of compassion and be honest.

4. The fourth and final stage of R.A.I.N., *non-identification*, is both a method and the result. If the first three stages worked, you're now dwelling in authentic presence. You're not identifying with the emotion or with any particular thoughts about the emotion, but your inner witness is just observing everything with a sense of openness and compassion. So there's no need to spin a narrative about what's happening inside your mind. There's no need to try to fix it with an agenda. Non-identification *is* authentic presence, actually. It's a sense of open awareness, peaceful and accommodating.

Conclusion

Really living authentically, in the present, through the presence of open, agenda-free awareness, is not a light switch that you turn on or off. It's a journey that requires persistent effort and courage. It is the continual expansion of the horizons of life. That only occurs if you keep applying yourself to the path again and again. The journey takes lot of guts.

It's easy to use meditation, yoga, and so on as accessories for our life. That way they can enhance our experience of ego. They can become another possession of ego. But they can't really touch us on a deeper level. And most of us don't want them to.

Authentic presence is not easy. It's no quick fix for the problems of life. All the wise seekers of the past are in agreement on that. But, if you stick with it, it can and will transform your life in every respect. Your mind will become better. You'll be more focused and intelligent. You'll carry your mood lightly, with a sense of humor. Strong emotions, when they come up, won't knock you off your seat, because you'll keep your awareness with steadiness and dignity. The way you treat others will be fair and compassionate. You will know how to treat them with empathy and respect. They will find you inspiring. They'll want to be around you.

So let me issue a challenge to you. I challenge you to set out on the path of authenticity. I challenge you to really surrender and open yourself up to the pulsing energy of life, without expectations or prefabricated goals. Go ahead and see what happens. I dare you.

**

If you enjoyed this book, then I'd like to ask you a favor. Would you be kind enough to share your thoughts and post a review of this book on Amazon? You could also let me know what you would like to see in future editions of this book

Your voice is important for this book to reach as many people as possible. The more reviews this book gets, the more people will be able to find it and enjoy the incredible benefits of meditation.

Preview of The Mindfulness Beginner's Bible

→ Available on Amazon
https://amzn.com/B01B6CD962

Chapter 1 - What is mindfulness?

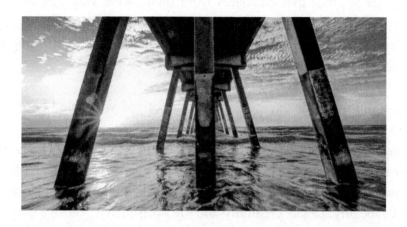

"Life is a dance. Mindfulness is witnessing that dance."
Amit Ray

Have you ever started eating a packet of chips and then suddenly realize that there is nothing left? This is one example of mindlessness that most of us experience on a daily basis. We, as humans often get so absorbed in our thoughts that we fail to experience what is happening right in front of us.

In modern society, most of us suffer from a condition called compulsive thinking. We have this hysterical inner voice that is constantly jumping from one thought to the next, obsessing about every little detail that could go wrong, complaining, comparing and criticizing everything and everyone. Sadly, most of us have become hostages to the whims of our minds, to the point where we even identify with the mind, thinking that we are our thoughts, when in reality we are the awareness behind our thoughts.

The moment you start observing your thoughts without identifying with them, you enter a higher level of consciousness beyond the mind and you reconnect with your true Self – the eternal part of you that is beyond the transient, ever-wavering physical realm.

Take a few seconds right now and become mindful of your hands. Feel the warmth that emanates from them. Rest your attention on every sensation in your hands. Feel your blood pulsing through them. Become one with your hands and notice the subtle tingling sensation as you become aware of them.

If you did this little exercise, I bet you noticed your mind becoming a bit more still. When you rest your attention on your body, you are living actively in the now. Awareness of the body instantly grounds you in the present moment and helps you awaken to a vast realm of consciousness beyond the mind, where all the things that truly matter - love, beauty, peace, creativity and joy - arise from.

Research has shown that we spend up to 50% of the time inside our heads - a state of mindlessness where we are continuously consumed by the chaotic impulses of our minds that are constantly thinking, ruminating the past and worrying about the future. Sadly, most people go through life in a walking haze, never really experiencing the present moment, which is our most precious asset.

Mindfulness is about being fully immersed into your inner and outer experience of the present moment. One of the best definitions of mindfulness is provided by the mindfulness teacher Jon Kabat-Zinn: "*Mindfulness means paying attention in a particular way; On purpose, in the present moment, and non-judgmentally.*"

Jon Kabat-Zinn breaks down mindfulness into its fundamental components: In mindfulness, our attention is held...

On purpose
Paying attention on purpose means intentionally directing your awareness. It goes beyond merely being aware of something. It means deliberately focusing your conscious awareness wherever you choose to, instead of being carried away in the perpetual storm of your thoughts.

Secondly, our attention is plunged...

In the Present Moment
The mind's natural tendency is to wander away from the present and get lost in the past or the future. Mindfulness requires being in complete non-resistance to the present moment.

Finally, our attention is held...

Non judgmentally
In mindfulness there is no judgment, there is no labeling, there is no resistance and there is no attachment. You simply observe your thoughts, feelings and sensations as they arise without ever energizing with them. As soon as you realize that you are not your thoughts, but the observer behind your thoughts, they will immediately lose power over your.

Mindfulness goes beyond basic awareness of your present experience. You could be aware that you are drinking tea, for example, however mindfully drinking tea looks very different. When you are mindfully drinking tea, you are purposefully aware of the entire process of drinking tea – you feel the warmth of the cup, the subtleties in smell and taste of the tea, the sensation of heat as you press your lips against the cup... – you intentionally immerse yourself in every single sensory detail that makes up the experience of drinking tea, to the point where you completely dissolve into the activity.

Mindfulness is about maintaining the intention of being completely plunged into your experience, whether it is drinking tea, breathing or doing the dishes. You can bring mindfulness to virtually any activity in your life.

Chapter 2 - The Power of the Present Moment

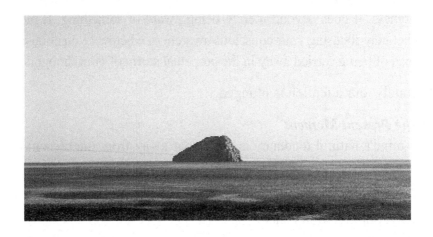

"I have realized that the past and future are real illusions, that they exist in the present, which is what there is and all there is."
Alan Watts

When you think about it, the present moment is the only moment that really exists. The past and the future are merely persistent illusions – the past is obviously over, and the future hasn't happened yet. As the saying goes, "*Tomorrow never comes*". The future is merely a mental construct that is always around the corner.

Even when you dwell on the past or worry about the future, you're doing so in the present moment. At the end of the day, the present moment is all you and I have, and to spend most of our time outside the present means we are never truly living. Spiritual leader Eckhart Tolle puts it beautifully: "*People don't realize that now is all there ever is; there is no past or future except as memory or anticipation in your mind.*"

However, most people spend most of their waking time imprisoned within the walls of their own thoughts, usually in regret of the past or in fear of the future, which are two ways of not living at all.

The present is the only moment in our lives where we have complete control over our destiny. We can decide our course of action only in the now – we can make a new friend, start a new business, get back to the gym, decide to stop smoking... The present is the only moment where your creative power can be exercised; it is the only place where you have full control over your life. Embracing the present moment is the only way to live a happier, healthier and more fulfilling life. As Buddha said, *"The secret of health for both mind and body is not to mourn for the past, worry about the future, or anticipate troubles, but to live in the present moment wisely and earnestly."*

The biggest obstacle that keeps us from living in the present moment is the mind. Embracing mindfulness is a journey that requires practice and dedication, but it is a process that will inevitably lead you to a much happier and more fulfilling life where every moment is lived to the fullest. Here are 8 steps to start living in the present moment:

Practice non-resistance

The first step towards living in the present is learning to live in acceptance. You must learn to accept your life as it is today, rather than wish it was any other way. You must come into complete non-resistance with your current experience of life. By letting go of the hold the past has over you, you free your mind from unproductive thoughts and you reclaim the present moment. As Eckhart Tolle says, *"Accept - then act. Whatever the present moment contains, accept it as if you had chosen it. Always work with it, not against it."*

Focus on the Now

In order to live in the present moment, you must focus on what you are doing in the now, whatever it may be. If you are doing the dishes, then do the dishes. If you're eating dinner, then eat dinner.

Don't view the seemingly mundane activities in your life as nuisances that you hurry to get out of the way. These moments are what our lives are made up of, and not being present in them means we are not truly living.

Don't take your thoughts too seriously

Identification with the mind is the root of much unhappiness, disease and misery in the world. Most people have become so identified with their mental chatter that they become slaves to their own compulsive thoughts. Being unable to stop thinking and means we are never living in the present moment. When you learn to observe your thoughts as they come and go without identification, you step away from the chaotic impulses of the mind and you ground yourself in the now.

Meditate

You don't have to meditate to be mindful, but research has shown that engaging in a regular meditation practice has a spillover effect on the rest of your life. When you meditate you essentially carry the state of stillness and awareness that you experience during your meditation session into the rest of your day. Meditation is practice for the rest of your life.

Pay attention to the little things

Notice the seemingly insignificant things around you. Pay attention to nature for example. Notice the greenery around you - be grateful for every tree, every plant, every flower and realize that you could not survive without their presence. Go through your life as if everything is a miracle. From the majestic rising of the sun, to the chirping of birds outside your window, to the fact that your heart is beating every single second – life is truly a miracle to behold when you immerse yourself in the present moment.

Do one thing at a time

Multitasking is the opposite of living in the now. When your attention is divided between several tasks like eating, driving, making a phone call, you cannot fully experience the present moment. Studies have shown that people who multitask take about 50% longer to complete a task with a 50% larger error rate. To be more mindful, you must become a single-tasker. When you're eating, just eat. When you're talking to people, just talk to them. Develop the habit of being completely immersed into whatever you're doing. Not only will you be more efficient, but you'll also be more alive.

Don' try to quiet your mind

Living in the present moment does not require any special effort. The present moment is already at your fingertips. There is no need to expand energy to empty your mind. In mindfulness there is no stress, no struggle and no effort because you are not trying to force anything – you are in complete non-resistance to your current experience of life.

Stop worrying about the future

Worry takes you out of the present moment and in the future into an infinite world of possibilities. You cannot worry about the future and simultaneously live in the present moment. Instead of worrying about things that may or may not happen, spend you time preparing to the best of your ability and let go of the rest. Worrying won't change the future, but it will definitely elevate the cortisol levels in your body and drain you of your vital energy.

→ Available on Amazon
https://amzn.com/B01B6CD962

→ <u>Available on Amazon</u>
https://amzn.com/B01H417582

Chapter 1: Worldview

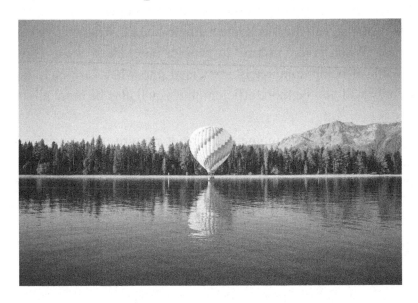

1. Suffering and Neurosis

According to Buddhism, before it makes sense to actually get down to the nitty gritty of working with your mind through the practice of meditation, you have to have a basic understanding of what you're doing and why. Otherwise, any kind of practice you do will lack direction. You will have a lot of doubt and confusion about what you're doing, which will easily knock you off the path.

The reason for searching for a spiritual path (or some kind of therapeutic practice, if you prefer) in the first place is that we feel somehow dissatisfied with our current situation. We're restless and want to change something, so we go looking for solutions.

That may sound very general, but so is our sense of unease and dissatisfaction. This very general sense of unease is what Buddhism calls *dukkha* or suffering.

The original meaning of *dukkha* is a kind of bad wagon wheel. The hole in the middle of the wheel, through which the axle is fitted, is off-center. So when you're riding in the wagon, the ride is bumpy and uncomfortable. That's because something is off. The wheel is not well-made. So the idea behind *dukkha* is that something is off in our minds. We're not crazy, necessarily, but we are looking at things sideways. We're off-center, and that creates the experience of suffering.

The Buddha's insight into the nature of suffering is that our experience of suffering has a cause. The cause of suffering is neurosis, which consists of passion, aggression, and confusion.

- *Passion* is the way the mind goes after some object of desire and moves us to action to get that object. There's a sense that we want to draw the object into our territory, to possess it and make it part of our little treasure hoard—especially if the object makes us feel good. So rather than let things be naturally, we try to draw them into the sphere of our control so we can lay hold of the object of our pleasure it make it *mine*.

- *Aggression* is passion's opposite, or more like its evil twin. Whatever is unpleasant or makes us feel bad, we want to throw up a defensive wall to stop it; we want to launch an attack on it and destroy it. The instinct here is the same as in passion. We have our little territory, which we think of as *mine*, and we want to make sure nothing threatening can breach it. If it has already made its way past our defenses, we want to destroy it.

- *Confusion* means that we are insensitive and indifferent to the way things work. We don't notice how cause and effect work; we have no clue that when this happens, that happens, and we never learn from our mistakes— or, for that matter, figure out how to reproduce our successes. So we keep doing the things that, in the long run, make us unhappy, and we're too confused to do the things that will bring us happiness. We could also call this stupidity or cluelessness.

These three neuroses work together to produce the experience of suffering, *dukkha*. To understand how that is, it helps to consider the different kinds of suffering. We can divide it up three ways: plain old suffering, suffering of change, and background suffering.

- *Suffering of suffering* is any suffering of the obvious sort. You step barefoot on a piece of broken glass. Your boyfriend or girlfriend leaves you, which breaks your heart. You have to spend long hours on a tedious task at work, leaving you bored and restless. A stranger insults you, which makes you feel angry. You catch a cold.

Obviously, practicing Buddhism isn't going to remove the pain of a foot injury or alleviate the discomfort of a bad cough. But what it can do is transform the way you experience and respond to the many knocks and bumps and irritations of life. When we try to maintain ourselves and protect and/or enlarge our little territory, we just compound our suffering. Take that out of the picture, and pain becomes simple, direct, and manageable.

- The *suffering of change* means that one minute we're happy, and the next we're not. Because everything is constantly changing, we find it hard to hold on to anything. We cannot secure a cozy situation for ourselves, because situations always tend to fall apart. So you might enjoy a well-paying, steady job for years, but one day the company faces budget problems and you get laid off. Or you're enjoying an ice cream, but the scoop of ice cream falls out of the cone and lands in the dirt. Even before the situation changes, the suffering of change is already there, as a potential. Somewhere in the back of your mind, you know that things can't keep going so well forever.

- *Suffering of conditionality*, or background suffering, is always present. It means that, because whatever experience you have is colored by passion, aggression, and confusion, it already contains some subtle level of suffering in it—always. This suffering is pervasive and subtle and lurks in the background. It is a nagging sense of anxiety that leads you to try to maintain and protect yourself and your territory, to create a little island of immunity in the confusing and threatening flux of life.

2. Further complications

Once we're already stuck in the pattern of churning out neurotic states of mind, the process has a way of keeping itself going in perpetual motion. One of the Buddha's key insights, which was revolutionary at the time, is that mental states are like anything else: they come about due to causes and conditions. A seed planted in the ground, when it meets with the right conditions of water, sunlight, and good soil, first sprouts and then grows into a fully sized plant.

Likewise, the life of the mind—the inner world of our experience—also follows a regular pattern of cause and effect, something that Buddhism calls *dependent arising*. When you set up the right conditions for *dukhha*, then you will have the experience of *dukkha*. And when you set up the right conditions for eliminating that suffering and experiencing freedom, you will have the experience of freedom from *dukkha*.

The Buddhist understanding of dependent arising is that the first event in this process causes a cascade of events that leads to the last one, and the last one then feeds back into the first one and keeps things going in a cycle. This feedback loop just reinforces itself again and again, generating more and more distress and suffering. So the idea is to stop the feedback loop. Somehow or another, we have to remove the causes and conditions that keep the loop going.

The first link in this chain is fundamental *ignorance*. This means that at the root of our problem is a mistaken thought or belief, a lack of the right kind of knowledge. Specifically, we don't have knowledge of impermanence and non-self (more on that later), which are the basic nature of reality. Because we get the basics so wrong, we get just about everything else wrong, also. So ignorance is the true origin of our distress.

Ignorance lays the foundation for our *mental conditioning*, which is the way our minds are predisposed to certain kinds of action. Some people are predisposed to certain bad habits—smoking, for example. They are already *conditioned* to act that way. They are conditioned by their own previous actions, and by their ignorance about the basic nature of things.

So, to continue the example, if we understand the nature of impermanence, then we'll know that the pleasure that comes from smoking is fleeting, that it puts us at risk for certain kinds of illness and hastens the approach of death. If we understand non-self, we won't be disposed to self-identities that reinforce this habit: *I am a smoker, I smoke because X, Y, and Z,* and so on. Conditioning includes everything from this simple example to full-blown psychological complexes.

Ignorance and conditioning are mostly subconscious. We're not really aware of them most of the time, but there they are anyway, influencing everything we think, say, and do. They provide the condition and background for *consciousness*, which is the next link on the chain. Here when Buddhism talks about consciousness, it doesn't mean a passive awareness of the world. This consciousness has a forward momentum and projects you into new situations, always pushes you into new kinds of action.

The way Buddhism thinks about things is a little different. Our usual intuition is that we have a body and mind and that consciousness is an operation of our mind. But the Buddhist way of thinking always puts *experience* front and center. So, because our experience of consciousness is very basic, it is considered as the foundation for our experience of *body and mind.* Any knowledge we have of our bodies, or of having this or that mental state, comes through our conscious experience of being a human in a body, our conscious experience of having a mind with all its thoughts, emotions, etc.

From this experience of body-and-mind comes our *sensory* experience. Consciousness moves forward, into the experience of body-and-mind, and then out towards the world, which it perceives in terms of sight, sound, smell, taste, and touch. Let's add another sense: consciousness is also aware of an inner world of thoughts and emotions, a mental sense.

69

The world "out there" comes into *contact* with the senses. And, from our point of view, this contact is either pleasant, unpleasant, or neutral—that is, it has a *feeling* to it. Now, whether an experience is pleasant or unpleasant is highly individual and based on each person's conditioning. Many people are fond of cucumbers, but I personally can't stand them.

Based on that pleasant or unpleasant feeling tone of an experience, another link in the chain comes up: *craving*. The word "craving" is a bit misleading here, because it refers not just to wanting things, but also to wanting to get rid of some other things. For that reason, really wanting to get a massage is craving, and so is being irritated by a mosquito bite.

The mind first craves, then it reaches or *grasps*. Because we crave something so badly, we try to grasp it, and stick to it like meat to a hot frying pan. So, with craving, we have a desire, while with grasping, we act on that desire.

Here, if we're good meditators, we have an opportunity to introduce a break in the feedback loop. A kind of space occurs between craving and grasping, a split-second gap in the chain of events. With a disciplined mind, it's possible to open that gap and stop the chain of events before they reach grasping. You have to be ready for it, because once you're grasping, it's already too late.

Grasping just fuels the fire and leads to further developments. Because we took action, our situation changes, grows, expands. The movement towards new states of being, fueled by the action of grasping, is called *becoming*, and becoming leads to the maturation of new situations and states of being, called *birth*.

But because of impermanence, whatever is born has to die. Any new situation we experience will start to fall apart and finally expire. This last stage is called *aging and death*. It is the true fruit of ignorance. Decay and death cause us tremendous suffering *because* of our ignorance of impermanence and non-self. We try to freeze or solidify our ever-changing experience, including our experience of self. We would like to believe that, underlying all this change, is a solid, consistent, unitary *I* that remains the same—in other words, a *self*. This habit is a deep feature of our psychology, and, as we'll see, it causes us a lot of grief.

→ Available on Amazon
   https://amzn.com/B01H417582

Made in the USA
Middletown, DE
16 December 2020

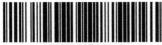